At 59 Ann Dredge had it all…

A blossoming young adult family, a growing business, excellent health and a happy marriage in its 38th year.

In excellent health, cycling 1000's of miles a year, playing the piano, Ann was reaching the stage of life where years of hard work was yielding rewards.

With both parents thriving in their mid-90's, Ann was looking forward to a rewarding 30 years.

All this came to a halt when she was told "You have early onset, atypical Alzheimer's. You are going to die. The only question is how soon."

For Ann and Peter, this was not an acceptable diagnosis. This was 2012. There must be a different outcome?

There was…

Peter Dredge

Beating Alzheimers: The Enemy At The Gate

Contents

"Never give in-
never, never, never,
in nothing great or small,
large or petty,
Never give in
except to convictions
of honour and good sense

Never yield to force;
Never yield to the apparently
overwhelming might of the enemy"

- Winston Churchill

"This is a war.
Alzheimer's is the
Enemy at the Gate.
Currently, we have no means
to defeat this enemy
but we can turn it away.
Hopefully, in time we'll have the resources
for a complete victory."

- Your humble author

Expert Prognosis

(The expectation we faced)

- Ann has severe Dementia of Alzheimer's-type, end stage.

- Ann's brain disorder is in its terminal phase.

- Ann requires physiotherapy and nursing work to intensively manage her developing contractures.

- Ann is very unlikely to survive the next twelve months; I would estimate her prognosis is three to six months.

- The key issues are regarding problematic swallowing, poor respiratory effort, recurrent urinary infections which have been reported, fixed contractures with the probability of developing pressure areas.

- There is no specific treatment to reverse this pathology, and she requires intensive supportive care in a dementia unit.

Consulting Neurologist's Report

September 19 2017

Foreword

Why the book?

You're likely affected by Alzheimer's. Directly or indirectly. If not, you will be.

First, a few facts:

In 1906 a German doctor, Alois Alzheimer, linked loss of cognitive function to brain damage in his patient, Auguste Deter. For the 5 years prior to Auguste's death, Dr Alzheimer charted her decline.

Subsequent autopsy revealed damage to her brain — an accumulation of detritus and plaques, subsequently identified as 'Sooty Tangles' and 'Amyloid Plaques'.

Since that time though, over more than a century, very little progress has been made with treating this 'disease'. No other field of medicine can claim *so little* advancement in 110-plus years.

Today around 40 million people in the world display Alzheimer's symptoms, a figure expected to increase to 150 million globally by 2050. To put it in another perspective, by 2050 nearly *half of people over age 85* will display Alzheimer's symptoms.

Statistically, this will arguably likely either be you, or the person next to you. Sufferer or caregiver — one of these is your likely future.

Alzheimer's is fast becoming the biggest medical, social, financial challenge of this century.

So why the book?

Over the past ten years, Ann and I have travelled a journey...

From **confusion** to **despair**

From despair to **knowledge**

From knowledge to **action**

From action to **hope**

From hope to **success.**

It's an ongoing journey — it will continue for the rest of our lives. We'll never drop our guard because, although the enemy has retreated, it is still out there.

As our journey turned from despair to hope, as Ann's condition turned from decline to recovery, it became ever more important to share our story.

We'll show you how to start your journey

We're not unique. You can do this too.

My mission is to show you where to begin. To chart our journey so you can start yours, hopefully avoiding the pitfalls we've experienced.

Tip: In this book, I'll offer you ten rules to help you on your way.

Introduction
&
Background

Ann's consulting neurologist had delivered a hopeless prognosis. I refused to accept it.

Every year many thousands of people are told that they, or a loved one, have Alzheimer's disease. They're told by their medical professionals that nothing can be done: no miracle cure exists.

"There is no magic pill," they say. "You're going to decline, then die. The only variable being the speed of the decline."

Their best suggestion? "You'd best get your affairs in order."

This is not necessarily true

They're right, no miracle cure exists. However, a large body of credible published research tells us:

Alzheimer's is an inflammatory response
It makes sense to investigate what is *causing* this response.

Alzheimer's is not so much a disease as a range of symptoms with many possible causes
Today, mainstream medical practice views Alzheimer's much as 19th century medicine viewed 'the fever'. They saw it as a single problem, whereas we now know that 'the fever' was a set of reactive symptoms to any number of possible complaints.

We've long regarded the practitioners of that day as hopelessly ill-informed and misguided. And yet – despite having 110 years to get it right – today's mainstream Alzheimer's medical practitioners seem blindly obsessed with finding a "silver bullet" cure. It's an impossible, naïve dream. A dream killing many people.

What does this mean?

Given the complexity of the symptoms, it means **the search for a 'single' cure may be hopelessly misguided.** Twenty-five years of research and many millions spent on drug trials have led to a mere handful of mostly ineffective medications being registered.

It's likely that no other field of medicine has failed so dismally to gain a toehold with such a widespread condition. Many once intractable medical conditions are now showing rapidly increasing survival and remission rates. Not so for mainstream medicine in dealing with Alzheimer's.

Credible research going back many years has built a large body of knowledge pointing towards effective treatments and preventative practices. Practices currently demonstrating arrest and reversal of Alzheimer's symptoms.

Most of this knowledge is coming from leading universities with independent research teams driven by good science. Not by the pursuit of an elusive and unrealistic desire to find a simple (and lucrative) solution.

Over the last 18 months I've come to realise that the biggest enemy is the palliative health and disability residential care system. A system which firmly believes there is no alternative to an early inevitable demise for Alzheimer's sufferers.

The health practitioners hold a strong belief that they are very smart people. Consequently their opinion that Alzheimer's can't be arrested or reversed must be valid. Regardless of the strong evidence to the contrary. Rather than question these beliefs in the face of new evidence, they determinedly set out to destroy the credibility of anyone who challenges their orthodoxy.

With such beliefs and huge vested interest, deprivation of hope and an early demise is inevitable. For the palliative dementia care industry, this is very profitable.

It's not so much that the system is operated by cynical people. It's more that a firm, misguided belief system is driving a juggernaut with huge momentum. The residential care operators literally do not want to know that credible alternatives exist.

And yet, **right now, teams are treating people experiencing early stage Alzheimer's symptoms**

with high levels of success. This is not a cure, but it does arrest the decline and supports recovery of lost function.

True, non-compliance with these programs, once established, leads to a reoccurrence of former symptoms and continued cognitive decline. But when your previous success rate is zero, demonstrated success rates in excess of 80% over an 18 year period should be of intense interest.

You'd think a small but reliable sample of that magnitude is way more significant than hundreds of samples with zero success. Looking in the wrong direction and repeatedly analysing your results is not only dimwitted, it's bordering on delusional.

By chronicling our journey, I hope to illustrate what we're up against and show you a way forward.

Let's look for some signposts to help guide our way:

- Alzheimer's is a rapidly increasing problem, showing up ever earlier.

- The symptoms are virtually unknown in some cultures, especially those with simple traditional diets.

- Indications are that lifestyle is a major factor.

- All of us will experience Alzheimer's either personally or in someone near to us.

Before I begin . . .

Before introducing you to Ann's story, I want to ask you to keep FOUR things in mind:

1. If we step away from viewing Alzheimer's as a disease, and view it as an inflammatory response, then we can start to look for causative factors. As with 'fever' in the 19th Century, we know it is the body's response to any, or some, of a number of factors. Although each factor may prove individually treatable, mainstream medical practice has the 'fever' view of Alzheimer's. To succeed, we can't share the mainstream view.

2. Dietary changes will be necessary. A **key factor** in many Alzheimer's sufferer's brains is, they don't metabolise glucose at all well.

3. Beating Alzheimers won't be easy. The reality is that life isn't easy, despite our desire for it to be so. Don't ever ask the question "Why is this happening to us?" It will uselessly waste time. Time is not your friend.

4. Most importantly... You the carer, are going to need to 'break the mould' to save your loved one. If you don't, they'll die before they should. It's a huge responsibility.

Chapter 1

Ann

A High-achieving Super Mum

What Ann saw in an underachieving, troublemaking high school boy like myself remains a mystery. To me at least.

We first met as 15 year-olds at Rutherford High School, Auckland, New Zealand, in 1967. Ann's first recollection of me was my ejection from our maths class for refusing to do homework. (Mind you, the homework covered topics I'd mastered a year earlier!)

We became good friends throughout our high school years. Ann was my opposite, being a high achiever with many extracurricular activities including sports, gymnastics, music and theatre. She was also unusual in our day, being one of the few young women studying sciences. Ann had the distinction of being the only girl in our senior high school physics class.

In 1970 Ann departed for Otago University, at the other end of the country. She studied for a degree in biochemistry. I stayed on to study, irresolutely, at Auckland University.

Upon Ann's return to Auckland in 1972, we came together as lovers and partners, living together until marrying in 1974. Living together was a scandalous occurrence in that early-seventies New Zealand.

From 1974 to 1976 Ann supported me as I completed my university degree and teacher's studies. She'd already completed her degree in cell biology.

In 1977 Ann completed her postgraduate studies as a librarian. She had the distinction of being that oh-so-rare creature of the time, a *librarian* with a *science* degree. Her career involved work in university medical and science libraries. She was a pioneer in online search engine operation, a brand-new field in the late 1970's.

Ann supported me whilst I worked full time building a 32' steel yacht in the early 1980's. She had the added 'pleasure' of spending her spare time also working on the boat. Leaving New Zealand in '83, we sailed *Aeolia II* to Washington DC, via Australia, South Africa, Brazil and the Caribbean.

We started our family in Washington DC with Nicholas, born there in 1985. Rachel and Sam following after our return to New Zealand in 1986. Three children in just over three years …

Over the next 25 years, Ann carried out her 'Super Mum' role. Working for much of the time, she was the multi-tasking miracle worker. She held the family together whilst I worked on various businesses which tended to demand more time than they should have.

Still, we found time to share recreational road cycling, which we very much enjoyed both on our own and with organised groups.

So this was Ann, come 2010...

Super mum to a young adult family of three

Wonderful wife, partner and lover

Veteran sailor

Accomplished pianist

Super-fit cyclist

Highly competent administrator for
our new, successful life insurance business

In short: a vibrant, healthy 57 year old woman with the prospect of many full and happy years ahead.

Chapter 2

The First Signs

**Things weren't quite right.
Something was a little … off-key**

In retrospect, it's possible to notice signs as early as 2008. Ann, then 55, was helping me with the administration of a financial planning service to which I was contracting at the time. I remember Ann being a little — slow — organising client files, a task she breezed through before.

By 2010, after we had started our life insurance brokerage, it was clear that Ann was struggling with organising paperwork: Date sequencing was a particular problem; our apartment, also our home office, was covered in drifts of paper which seemed to move but never settle into a file. Insurance was a paper-intensive business at that time!

I was away from home running a remote office 3 - 4 nights a week. I didn't really grasp the extent of the growing problem.

Together, we decided that something was not right. Ann's doctor, a woman, told her that the slowness was just a result of menopause and she should get used to it. Not a useful response, and a good indicator of advice and events to come.

We sidelined that doctor and started doing our own research. Our first suspect was 'menopausal fuzzy brain' Approaching a hormone specialist medical practice, we expected thorough analysis of Ann's hormone levels and perhaps some pointers towards what was going wrong.

Our experience was less than satisfactory. The expected analysis turned out to be a vague trial and error sequence to see whether an individual hormone made any difference. There was no improvement after some months and, worse, no apparent willingness by the practice to look at Ann as a whole person with possible issues outside their blinkered view.

Through 2010 and 2011, Ann was finding driving to be a challenge. She told me that navigation had become hard. She would find herself at a place without any recollection of how she got there. Luckily our children were now driving, so many journeys were taken with a family member driving.

On our cycling outings, I noticed that Ann tended to wander off the road shoulder in front of approaching vehicles. Not a healthy trend for a cyclist! Friends also noticed and spoke of their worry about Ann's road-keeping habits.

It was soon late-2011. We'd changed medical practices, Ann's new doctor had her complete the Mini Mental Status Examination (MMSE) and the test indicated that Ann had some troubles with visual spatial perception. For example, she struggled to draw a clock face with the hands at 10 minutes past 5 o'clock. A referral was made to a consulting neurologist.

Early in 2012, Ann took her first and last drive in a new car we'd purchased for her 3 months earlier. She became lost very easily and no longer felt competent to drive safely. Then in June of that year, Ann was diagnosed with early onset "atypical" Alzheimer's disease.

Chapter 3

Our Early Medical Journey

Much money is wasted; Ann is invited to become part of someone's science project.

Following our doctor's good detective work, we visited a consulting neurologist. The neurologist assessed Ann and referred her her to another neurologist, who specialised in Alzheimer's disease. This is where our experience began to get very strange indeed!

Following the advice of the Alzheimer's specialist, we paid for a MRI scan of Ann's brain. I(Although MRI scans are available free of charge in New Zealand's public health system, there can be some delay in scheduling an appointment so we elected to pay a private clinic for an immediate scan.)

Our understanding was that Ann's scan was *urgent*. It was needed to assist diagnosis and establish a a course of action to help Ann's condition. More than a decade into the 21st century, we had no suspicion that a common problem like Alzheimer's was still considered a medical dead-end.

With the expensive scan in hand, we met with the specialist again. Expecting a way forward, we felt that we now had some hope. I mean, knowledge is power, right?

Not at all!

Instead, we were **told** —

Ann's right parietal lobe showed deterioration with some gaps apparent between sections of her forebrain; the section of the brain responsible for sequencing and visual-spatial organisation, amongst other tasks.

A psychological evaluation was required to get a close analysis of Ann's functionality

No effective treatment was available to arrest or reverse the process. We "learned" that ALL people with Alzheimer's will decline, then die. The only variable is the rate of decline.

One of the very few drugs of possible benefit was Donezipil, but it was of questionable effectiveness and could have terrible side effects.

We needed to keep a good record of Ann's decline to help further Alzheimer's research. Including further scans.

And, we were posed a question: **"Oh, by the way, can we have your brain when you've finished with it?"**

At this point, we had no real option but to accept the terrible, apparently inevitable, outcome mapped out for us. As happens to so many, we went away to consider how we'd spend our remaining time together.

Before the 'lights came on' for us later in our medical journey, Ann endured hugely stressful, upsetting psychological testing. There's no joy in documenting what you've lost and will "never recover" according to the experts.

Significantly, the psychologist noted Ann's *awareness* of her functional loss — very unusual for people with Alzheimer's symptoms.

She also underwent another, expensive, 'urgent' scan some months later. The purpose of this was to establish a rate of decline.

After all of this, Ann was invited to join a specific research project which was to map her's and others' decline — the purpose apparently was to see whether some useful data could be gleaned. Effectively a doomed "control" group.

At no stage in this process was there mention of even the existence of possible alternative credible schools of thought about treating Alzheimer's disease. Up to this point our experience could easily be summarised as:

"Ann, you're going to die. The only question is how soon. By the way, how would you like to be part of our jolly old science project?"

1. Pete's First Rule for Beating Alzheimer's

No neurologists! Taking an Alzheimer's sufferer to a neurologist and expecting an improvement is as effective as asking an electrician to fix your toilet.

A neurologist will carry out minimal testing, happily chart your loved one's condition and then tell you nothing can be done. Once you understand the breadth of the problem, you'll also understand that, at least at this time of writing, a neurologist is of little practical use.

In fact, it has an opposite effect: In your further dealings with the medical world, the diagnosis of Alzheimer's, whether rightly or wrongly assessed, will carry weight and become an *obstacle* to effectively treating the symptoms.

To call it a diagnosis is misleading and glorifies an abysmal blindness to good science and effective diagnostic practice. The very word 'Diagnosis', a word which carries weight and life-altering (often even life-shortening) implications, absolutely requires three things. To my mind at least:

- The doctor knows in detail what the condition is

- The causes are well known and documented

- A pathway to treatment — or at least amelioration of symptoms — can be established, or will be at some point, hopefully soon.

For us, it was a 'fail' on all 3 counts! What were we really getting? It's simple ... merely **a description of symptoms** ... nothing more.

If you're a doctor or neurologist reading this, are you offended? Good. You should be doing a lot better.

Chapter 4

The Lights Come On

We take control and hunt for alternatives

The first sign of hope came when we stumbled across Dr Mary Newport's excellent book, *Alzheimer's Disease, What if There was a Cure?* Dr Newport reported on the cognitive improvements her husband Steve underwent when fed a significant amount of coconut oil. The oil being mixed with its derivative, medium-chain triglyceride (MCT) oil.

The book pointed us to the dietary advantages of coconut oil as an aid to cognitive function for Alzheimer's sufferers. The key message being that Alzheimer's-afflicted brains are insulin-resistant. *Feeding an Alzheimer's sufferer a normal carbohydrate rich diet starves their brain.*

I'll try to explain: A brain cell has two energy 'doors'. The 'front door' lets in glucose as an energy source. The 'back door' lets in *ketones* as an alternative energy source. Ketones are our body's emergency energy source in times of hardship, and are typically drawn from our body fat.

For Alzheimer's sufferers, that front 'glucose' door is either closed, or only partially open. The brain cannot get the energy it needs from a normal western diet rich in simple carbohydrates. If it doesn't get the energy it needs, the brain *literally starves*. Obviously, this has poor implications for functionality and brain health.

To alleviate this problem, an alternative source of energy is required: Ketones.

So how can you do this? In two ways. Firstly, by keeping the body 'Ketogenic' so the body is in a mode where it is accessing its fat for energy. (Our bodies typically are not in this mode, we love carbohydrates too much!)

Secondly, supplying the body with that fat-rich food that metabolises instantly into ketones — which then become available for the brain to use as an energy source.

So — what did we do, and what did it achieve?

Firstly, we continued with Ann's Ketogenic diet — low in starchy carbohydrates with no sugar. This was a dietary regime we'd maintained off and on since discovering Dr Barry Sear's Zone Diet in the late 90's. We'd found weight control easier, and athletic performance was enhanced.

Most notably, we started supplementing Ann's diet with 120ml (4 fl oz) of a 40% coconut oil and 60% MCT oil mix daily. Generally taken with food and hot drinks.

What happened?

Ann had been having **daily occurrences of full body twitches for an hour or more after waking**. Distressing to watch. These disappeared and have rarely reoccurred. On the odd occasion they did, a dose of oil mix cured the problem.

Ann had been having trouble dressing herself for the daily cycle rides on our tandem bike. As winter approached, she needed to don more than 15 items of clothing. **Almost immediately, her difficulties ceased**.

Even now, Ann still receives a significant dosage of the oil mix. Its absence has been shown to have deleterious effects.

In effect we had turned back the clock, but that's all we'd achieved so far. Luckily there was more to follow.

Early in 2016, a friend pointed us to an article, published November 2015, in a national magazine *The Listener*. The article reported on the work being undertaken by Dr Dale Bredesen of UCLA — the University of California Los Angeles.

Over the preceding 30 years Dr Bredesen had developed the ReCODE diagnostic and treatment protocol. The protocol had shown high levels of success with Alzheimer's mice since the year 2000. The *Listener* article covered an initial human trial reported in *Ageing Magazine*, September 2014.

This first human trial — on ten subjects — started in 2012. The results showed an arrested decline and reversal of symptoms in nine out of the ten patients. Six of the subjects had ceased working owing to cognitive impairment. All six returned to work. The tenth subject had advanced Alzheimer's and did not respond to the treatment protocol.

Bredesen's protocol, being multi-faceted, seemed credible, especially as it acknowledged the huge complexity of the problem. ReCODE came at Alzheimer's symptoms from a number of angles. This aligned with our feeling that Ann's issues were complex and defied simplistic answers.

We felt at that time, in 2016, it defied credibility that the whole medical and scientific community had made zero progress on sorting out the Western World's largest approaching health problem. It seemed Bredesen was heading in the right direction but, unfortunately, at that point the treatment protocol wasn't available outside the United States. What to do?

Well, Bredesen had listed a number of supplements from which he had selected all or some to administer to each member of his trial group. So we tried this — a difficult task requiring a twice-daily intake of more than a dozen supplements, including some very large pills. Ann, as always, was an absolute trouper, suffering this onerous task without complaint.

This seemed to work. Another uptick in performance. Formerly a voracious reader, Ann had become unable to read more than a handful of pages at a time, which were often read repeatedly. Quickly, she again began reading large sections of her book in single sessions.

However, this uptick didn't last too long — fate stepped in to derail her progress.

Two steps forward, one step back

Late in 2015, with the support of Assistance Dogs New Zealand, we had been privileged to receive New Zealand's first fully trained Alzheimer's assistance dog. Lexus, a two year old Labrador cross, was to assist with Ann's emerging mobility problems.

A major issue for us had been Ann losing sight of me when we were out and about. She would easily become lost; I had only to turn my back and she would be gone. Although her eyesight was apparently normal, her condition caused her to lose sight of me from even a close distance. A real and distressing problem when shopping or walking in busy public spaces.

The generosity of the many people who donated through a crowd funding campaign was both heartening and humbling. The cost of NZ$20,000 was raised in three weeks, and Lexus joined us December 2015. She was a huge blessing with her ability to keep Ann on track when we were out together. Having being trained for two years, Lexus was extremely intelligent with a large toolbox of skills to draw on for Ann's needs.

Perhaps as important, Ann had been continually losing parts of her life. This was the first time that she had *gained* something exclusively hers.

We spent the Christmas Holiday period, January 2016, getting to know and bond with Lexus. During this time we travelled to the far south of New Zealand to buy a Winnebago Class A motorhome. The thousand mile trip home was great fun and a highlight for us as a couple.

A day after our return home, disaster struck…

Lexus had one characteristic that defied her training and fine breeding. When delivered, her trainer told us that she was a "bit of a klutz". When working she was a model of calmness and skill. Removing her working jacket though, revealed a gambolling, clumsy, overgrown puppy!

Whilst galloping around in a nearby park, Lexus misjudged a run-by, designed presumably in her mind to closely miss my legs at high speed. Unfortunately I was talking to a neighbour and not paying attention — though that attention was gained as I heard a large crack and fell to the ground, my left knee smashed.

Eight days in hospital and two months on crutches made meeting Ann's increasing care needs very difficult. The mineral supplementation program fell victim to my recovery limitations. Then three months after this first setback, another eight day stay in hospital for me — this time with a ruptured appendix — further slowed Ann's program.

So 2016 was a year of increasing frustration. We *knew* that the medical methodology existed to possibly halt and reverse Ann's decline. However this wasn't available to us, and there was no indication of it becoming so.

Life events made it very hard to keep any semblance of organisation around Ann's requirements. Even such important needs as our regular tandem bike rides were not met.

We didn't know it then … but hope was on the horizon!

Chapter 5

Help arrives

Common sense and good
science come to the rescue

Once again fate intervened: Late in 2016, we were shown another article in the *Listener* Magazine: it said that the Bredesen Protocol for treating Alzheimer's was now available in New Zealand.

Dr Dave Jenkins, a New Zealand-trained medical general practitioner (GP) had been trained in the Bredesen Protocol, working directly with Dr Bredesen at the Buck Institute for Research on Ageing in California.

Dr Dave, as he's known, along with his partner, nutritionist Miki Okuno, had been appointed as the Bredesen Protocol Consultant for Australia and New Zealand. His role was to work with a patient's GP to oversee the necessary and complex testing. Then, following complex analysis of the test results, Dr Dave would liaise with the patient's GP to direct the treatment process. Typically Dr Dave would spend around a hundred hours per patient, annually.

Dr Dave has gained international recognition for his work in establishing a community development and medical charity in western Indonesia. He helped set up Surf Aid in 2000, after noticing the many children's graves in a local cemetery whilst on a surfing trip — one in ten children were dying before the age of five. Often from relatively easily treated illnesses: such as malaria and pneumonia. Surf Aid has since saved many lives and was a key aid provider after the 2004 Boxing Day tsunami.

We approached Dr Dave in January 2017. I well remember a Skype consultation with him as Ann and I sat in our RV beside an airfield during an airshow and the conversation was interrupted at times by low flying aircraft. (Although challenging, our lives aren't boring!)

By now, Ann was past early stage Alzheimer's, and — as far as I'm still aware — it was in that early stage where Bredesen and his team had, as at early 2017 at least, recorded their successes. Over the next three months Dr Dave and I discussed a possible course for Ann.

From January 2017 to March that year, I was also tasked with raising the necessary NZ$20,000 needed for the first year of Ann's treatment. Our resources were stretched as we now had no income apart from a meagre government pension and some consultancy work. Fortunately, family came to our aid and provided the necessary funding. New Zealand's free healthcare system wasn't able to help as the Bredesen treatment was viewed, rightly so at that point, as experimental. More on this later.

During these three months, Dr Dave and I had several discussions. His reservations related to Ann's now moderate and ever more rapidly advancing symptoms, but eventually I was able to persuade him we were better to try and fail than never to have tried.

I've already mentioned Ann's and my wedding vows.They were sworn in 1974 at the Hobsonville Airforce Base Church in Auckland with Ann's father, then an airforce chaplain, officiating. To us, "Until Death Us Do Part" was absolute. There was no "Or as long as it's still convenient" rider clause. Our wedding contract implied a heavy commitment to making sure that death would only come when all sensible avenues had been exhausted.

It was in early April 2017 that the real adventure began.

Chapter 6

Finding Out What's Really Wrong

Making huge progress... despite the medical profession; Further rules are established

After an exhaustive process of questionnaires and consultations, Dr Dave prepared comprehensive introductory information and made requests for in-depth testing.

Naïvely, I expected Ann's GP to be excited to hear that at least a *possibility* of hope existed for the many patients in his practice suffering from forms of dementia. I couldn't have been more wrong, which saddened me.

I organised a longer-than-usual consultation with the doctor, expecting a discussion around the comprehensive information the doctor had received from Dr Dave. The GP had some weeks to review the information — I wanted to be sure he had time to do some follow-up research. The information included reference to significant credible scientific research, with the trail — should the GP decide to follow it — going back some thirty years. This included more than two-hundred peer-reviewed papers published by Professor Bredesen alone, plus other artefacts.

None of the tests were out of the norm for general medical practice although, of necessity, they were wide ranging. Some thirty or more blood and urine tests were requested, but certainly none could possibly be construed as being harmful and all could be seen as providing helpful information. In my naïvety I expected the GP to be at least *interested* in the comprehensive information supplied and thought our meeting was to order the requested series of tests, as I'd explained in my correspondence to the doctor.

So... we had the consultation. Immediately the doctor launched into a long-winded dither, giving the many reasons not to do anything. With eyes dramatically rolled heavenwards, the doctor piously intoned the — unfortunately to become familiar — mantra of "First do no Harm". Translated by myself, Ann's impassioned activist, as a weak-kneed excuse: "First do Nothing, especially if I may have to exhibit some form of initiative, scientific enquiry and real concern for my patients' welfare". A theme so common that I now have a job description for new doctors: "Must have a functioning brain and spine."

This process had wasted a whole month, one that was precious and, at the time, I considered irretrievable. Ann was showing signs of accelerating deterioration. My last written communication with the doctor, though polite, was sharply pointed: I expressed my frustration with his lack of care for Ann's welfare, and suggested that he reflect on the fact that his dithering had dimmed her prospects considerably.

However, expressing frustration wasn't productive. And so I learned to multi task — let them know that you're disappointed whilst being well into the next step. Don't let them walk away scot-free.

So, what next?

After some Facebook requests which yielded nothing but the usual bevy of reactive, often strange, usually simplistic 'silver bullet' suggestions, I took to exploring Google to find out who could truly help.

By now, I'd learned a few things:

2. Pete's Second Rule for Beating Alzheimer's

Get the right doctor. The more a medical professional's website mentions "putting the patient first" the less likely they are to do so. The more salubrious the doctor's office, the less likely they are to be helpful.

Remember, we were only asking for a series of tests at this point, but these are required to be ordered by Ann's GP or other medical practitioner.

We approached a fancy 'alternative' (aka 'integrative' or 'holistic') medical practice in Auckland, New Zealand's biggest city, just over an hour's drive away. Naïvely expecting them to live up to their hype, we wasted a week or more supplying reams of information. Several follow-up calls later they said they couldn't help because it would all be too hard. This practice was, in my mind, a provider with a lack of a functioning spine.

Finally, desperate, I approached the second medical practice in our small town. The one with the small modest office in the main street, the 'socially aware' practice with patients definitely lower on the socio-economic scale — my inner white middle-class snob was being challenged.

Twenty-four hours later the tests were ordered, three days later the samples were taken.

It was May 2017 — we were on our way at last!

Chapter 7

Finally, a Result

Ann goes into care. We find out exactly what's happening — and that it's treatable

June 1st, 2017 — the day that things became really serious:

Ann had, for some time, been having private conversations with herself. Since the beginning of the year she'd also been having more-delusional episodes — which I had managed by giving her a good-sized sip of her coconut/MCT oil mix, either straight or in a hot drink. After drinking the oil — not a pleasant task — generally she would regain a relatively normal view of the world.

These episodes could be quite distressing for both of us. Ann was convinced I was someone very nasty and would berate me vigorously at times. Clearly she felt threatened and thus distressed. When asked who she thought I was, she'd reply "You're not my husband!". In her quieter moments I would joke that if she thought I was someone else, could it at least be someone nice?

Her conversations would often include a dialogue about a little girl who was in need of help and nobody would assist — this caused an episode which led to her being sedated and admitted to hospital. Thus began a decidedly rocky journey through the geriatric palliative care establishment, on which more later…

The test results combined with the details of Ann's progression led Dr Dave to suspect that Ann had a variant of 'Type 3' Alzheimer's in Bredesen's classification. This type describes Alzheimer's symptoms caused by environmental factors. As most cases described in the literature are the result of mould inhalation caused by leaky buildings, Bredesen has also called it 'Inhalational Alzheimer's'.

Unfortunately, the many tests carried out to date hadn't allowed for analysis of Ann's exact condition. To do this would require a travelling to a specialist lab in Melbourne, Australia — a three-hour flight. By this stage, late May 2017, it was clear that Ann was in no state to travel. We had reached an impasse.

For the next three months, during which Ann was in three rest homes and twice in hospital, Dr Dave and I racked our brains to get around the testing problem. The issue was the testing required a very short time to elapse between drawing the blood sample, and starting the analysis — a problem normally solved by having the samples drawn at the lab.

Dr Dave's considerable problem-solving skills won through. He negotiated a solution that allowed for samples to be collected in New Zealand and flown immediately to Australia.

The sample collection system was a thing of wonder. In early October 2017, Diana Hardwick Smith, a private phlebotomist, attended Ann at her (now fourth) rest home. Staggering in under the load of a desktop centrifuge, Diana set up shop. Collecting Ann's blood samples, she centrifuged them, packed them in ice and rushed them to the airport for transport to the lab.

Two weeks later we had our test results, and a result... Ann was suffering from Chronic Inflammatory Response Syndrome (CIRS) with one marker indicating possible Lyme disease causation. So, CIRS-PLS. PLS being Post Lyme Syndrome.

Ann's inflammatory markers were off the chart, literally. Her immune system was still reacting to the CIRS, generating a continual stream of biotoxins to deal with a problem now no longer present. These biotoxins had significantly damaged her brain.

Was this treatable? Yes. Dr Ritchie Shoemaker, with his USA-based team, had been working on the problem for the last 20 years. The treatment protocol, The Shoemaker Protocol, had been in use for the last 10 years with hundreds of case studies and many scientific papers documenting support for its efficacy. Shoemaker and his team had not only documented reversal of symptoms, but had also documented brain mass recovery in placebo trials.

Where had Ann contracted Lyme disease? New Zealand, to date, has no reported cases either in humans or animals — not because it doesn't exist (it may or may not) but it is not a notifiable disease in NZ. Hence no reported cases!

However, we'd holidayed in Fiji in 2007, and Fiji *does* have Lyme disease. One day we hired a taxi for a tour of the countryside around Nadi and the taxi driver took us to a couple of his family's farms. Both had various livestock around, clearly in less than optimum condition, most likely tick-infested. I have no recollection of Ann being bitten, or seeing the characteristic red ring, but this is not unusual as ticks often bite but don't attach themselves successfully and the ring can be hard to spot. Ann, at this point was in no state to comment.

What I can clearly remember, looking back, is that a few months after this Fijian escape, Ann started to struggle with paperwork — by then it was early 2008. Also clear was that toxic mould was unlikely to be an issue, because we had been living in very dry quarters at the time, on the third floor of a new beachfront apartment building.

Back to the main timeline: Between June and September 2017, Dr Dave and I had been discussing the likely causes of Ann's condition. Dr Dale Bredesen's paper on Inhalational Alzheimer's described a typical progression which mirrored Ann's, with early frontal lobe damage being the most significant physiological sign. The results of this damage showed up in visual-spatial tasks such as sequencing, organisation and visual acuity.

In Ann's case, paperwork, driving and descending stairs were early casualties of the condition. Another early symptom had been real difficulty in us staying together when out in the community. Supermarket shopping and walking together in crowded spaces had been an early problem. We would be walking together — then we weren't, Ann having lost sight of me whilst I was still nearby.

Dr Dave and I jointly decided that the best course was to treat Ann as if she had Type 3 Alzheimer's whilst we were organising the CIRS testing.

So we began the treatment journey.

Chapter 8

The Treatment Journey: Part I

We save Ann's life… in spite of her doctors

September 2017: Ann was no longer mobile, having been bed bound for two months. She had also been extremely agitated whenever awake, clearly of the impression that she was under attack.

Additionally, Ann had been dosed with very powerful anti-psychotic medication which has caused her physical harm. She no longer had the use of her left arm — a suspected side effect of the anti-psychotic drug, Haloperidol.

Ann had been assessed by a consulting neurologist as *unlikely* to live three months, *certainly* not six. We didn't expect her to see the family Christmas of 2017.

We had a strong suspicion that Ann had CIRS. The Shoemaker Protocol had given a clear, well proven, well documented treatment program. The first step of Shoemaker's program was to remove the biotoxins from Ann's system on a regular, daily basis.

And so, early in September 2017, we began treating Ann with three daily doses of Cholestyramine. Within two weeks, a miracle …

We first noticed that Ann had quietened down and appeared to be more aware of her surroundings. Friends and family came to visit, were recognised, warmly greeted. Ann was able to hold conversations and interject appropriately into discussions going on around her. She began to eat properly, recovering her formerly good appetite. And, she was able to report the need to use the toilet.

It was not to last. The rest home doctor was of the 'Alzheimer's can't be cured' school of thought, and was determined that her narrow view be reinforced by results rather than disproven. The drug required a medical prescription, so we secured a supply of Cholestyramine via an independent medical practitioner..

However, the recommendation via the Shoemaker Protocol was to have three daily administrations spread out around meals and medications. This required administration by the rest home medical staff, which in turn required the support of a doctor. We managed this for some time via Ann's external GP. However, it became harder in the face of opposition from the rest home GP.

Eventually, to keep the peace, we substituted activated charcoal for Cholestyramine. In addition, I naïvely thought that my administration of the new detox regime twice daily would suffice, instead of three times. To further complicate things, the activated charcoal caused bad constipation. I tried very hard to enlist the rest home doctor's support to get Ann's treatment back on track and to enable eventual further treatment, as recommended by Shoemaker.

October 2017: Ann's CIRS test results came in. I could now discuss with the rest home GP, a clearly-identified medical problem.

3. Pete's Third Rule for Beating Alzheimer's

Don't accept a closed mind.

"Stupid is as stupid does, Forrest" readily applies to many medical professionals.

Medical qualifications do not necessarily equate with an intelligent, open mind.

Mrs Gump's above-quoted wisdom (*Forrest Gump*) was to prove itself on a repeating basis.

By this point, I had learned that debating whether Alzheimer's is treatable or not was simply unproductive. Very similar to trying to convince a flat-earther they're misguided. People do not easily change an illogical position.

I now had definitive test results showing Ann was suffering from a very well-documented medical condition, with similarly well-documented treatment protocols to hand. The subsequent discussion with the rest home GP went thus:

Me: "Let's not worry about the Alzheimer's treatment debate. It isn't relevant as we now know what's wrong, Ann has CIRS. This is proven by her test results. Given these results, what's your suggestion for how we treat her?"

GP: "Nothing. I didn't order the tests".

Right on, Mrs Gump! In which particular universe would this doctor have *ever* ordered those tests? Certainly not this one!

4. Pete's Fourth Rule for Beating Alzheimer's

Get a doctor with a science background. Medicine and science are not necessarily good bedfellows.

Don't expect your doctor to pay attention to research documentation, no matter how good.

Check your doctor's qualifications. If they do not include a science degree and other experience prior to medical training, walk away.

A good rule of thumb to follow? Check your doctor's qualifications.

The doctors I've found most helpful generally had a science qualification and outside experience preceding their medical training. Modern doctors have become little more than glorified drug dispensing technicians, behaviour that has been reinforced by a treatment model which demands quick answers and simple solutions. It's an attitude to care that flies in the face of the current exponential growth of research and resultant medical knowledge.

You'll find the majority of doctors with only medical training will be dangerous to your loved one. You don't have the time to take the risk.

Ann's nascent treatment regime was failing. Add in a heatwave, plus confinement to a small, extremely hot, unventilated room at night, and Ann reverted to her previous state.

Six weeks followed with the rest home GP and attending psychiatrists attempting unsuccessfully to calm Ann with a range of questionable psycho-active drugs.

In mid-December 2017, Ann was admitted to the secure Psycho-geriatric wing of Auckland's North Shore Hospital.

5. Pete's Fifth Rule for Beating Alzheimer's

Avoid psychiatrists. They have cloth ears and wide ranging powers to take away your human rights.

Cloth ears? Yep, the listening skills of a stuffed toy. Ann's three months at this facility nearly killed her, twice. This period was a low point of Ann's experience, and she was most at risk during this hospital stay. Despite the excellent research and definitive medical results illustrating what we were up against, the ward's medical professionals decided, jointly, that:

Ann was in the late terminal stage of Alzheimer's. Death was imminent and I was deluded — unable to face the reality that Ann would die shortly.

With this mindset firmly in place, the psychiatrists set about proving themselves right.

I first knew we were in real trouble when the chief consulting psychiatrist drew himself up, puffed out his chest and said "I am a member of the Royal College of Psychiatrists and I know that Alzheimer's can't be treated." Apparently this was the end of the story.

My mindset? On the one hand I had him telling me, "Trust me, I'm a doctor and as such am incredibly smart and know Alzheimer's can't be treated". On the other hand I had international experts, their expertise backed-up by hundreds of research papers from top institutions, telling me otherwise. The second position seemed sensible to adopt, given my responsibilities to Ann.

Three months followed of ever-increasing sedation, which tended to make Ann more agitated when awake. Ann was sleeping a good twenty hours a day and when awake was stupefied, barely able to keep her eyes open or to recognise me.

I continually argued that her experience, when awake and being handled by care staff, was akin to a 'date rape' experience. She knew that something was happening that she hated and was unable to effectively resist or express her discomfort. The answer? More sedation, and so of course the problem worsened. When awake, Ann was continually agitated, shouting — sometimes screaming.

Even feeding Ann became hazardous to her health. Being barely awake, food and drink could find its way down her windpipe. This in turn could cause infection and bring on "aspiration pneumonia" — with which Ann had one serious bout and another near-miss. Again, the institutional view — this time that aspiration pneumonia was just an expected part of Ann's progression — didn't help. Only my insistence that Ann be fully treated for the pneumonia prevented her dying.

Aspiration pneumonia is a common cause of death for late-stage Alzheimer's patients

A convenient way to have them "shuffle off"?

At this stage Ann was assessed as being able to cope only with very mushy food and thickened liquids. Plates of food turned up which readily brought to mind the old adage '*Do* you eat it, or *have* you?' Pallid piles of watery mush were not in the least attractive. I tested the food and it tasted as bad as it looked. Ann was not eating much, the only way to get food into her was to shovel it in when she opened her mouth to shout or scream. The actual swallowing of the food happened by the process of it dissolving in her mouth as she further objected to its presence.

One day, the chief psychiatrist came to me, long-faced, and told me that Ann was no longer swallowing her food. This was a sure sign that she was entering the last stage of terminal Alzheimer's and that death was imminent. "Prepare yourself", was his advice.

No. I decided that we instead needed to credit Ann with some good sense. I had been suspicious all along that she was more aware than she appeared. What if she was objecting to the food?

She'd already said so! Rising from the depths of her sedation she'd occasionally shout "It's awful!" Ann had always possessed an excellent appetite, been a keen foodie and followed her family tradition of producing fantastic food.

I prepared her a chopped cucumber and tomato salsa. Immediately the problem went away. As she opened her mouth to scream, I inserted a spoonful of the salsa. Ann, as was her habit, opened her now full mouth to scream again... and stopped. She immediately started enthusiastically chewing. From that day, Ann's appetite improved. I prepared her lunch and dinner daily. So much for terminal late stage — 'Death by Mush' was the real problem!

The saga continued at the hospital. At times, I felt like a helpless participant at the Mad Hatter's Tea Party. Much time was spent by the psychiatrists trying to wrench me away from my 'delusion': The idea that Ann could survive and possibly recover to some degree. During one meeting I endured a psychiatrist screaming at me, "Alzheimer's can't be cured! You need to get used to the idea Ann's dying! It could be days away!" At this point Ann had a chest infection which, in their minds, would morph into pneumonia, bringing on the final, inevitable outcome.

Over the three months of her stay at the hospital, I attempted to preserve and progress Ann's recommended treatment regime. Not very effectively. The hospital would not co-operate in the reliable delivery of Ann's recommended medications and supplements, despite the thorough documentation provided. However, she showed signs of levelling out and had become a little calmer when awake.

In short, the doctors believed Ann was in the terminal late stages of Alzheimer's and were prepared to kill her to prove it. A harsh conclusion but we're in a milieu where an ill-informed view of Alzheimer's determined — and still determines — courses of action which if not guaranteed to kill a patient, certainly seem to aim towards an efficient early demise.

Again, in contrast Ann's caregivers and nurses were excellent: Caring and efficient.

Mid-March 2018: Ann had inconveniently defied the odds. The parts of the Shoemaker Protocol I'd been able to administer seemed to have calmed her and improved her state, albeit very slightly. We'd arrested her decline — a major victory at that point.

A rest home manager was visiting the ward, possibly looking for new clients. A harsh assessment? By this stage my normally positive view of people had been dented. The manager viewed Ann and assessed her as a suitable fit for the rest home she managed.

Shortly thereafter Ann was transferred to the rest home. We hoped she was now out of danger. The hospital psychiatrist's last gasp? Admonishment — I should not pressure the rest home to reduce Ann's current and stupefying levels of sedation. To ensure this, he had Ann's discharge summary specifically request that Ann's sedation not be altered by the rest home's attending doctor.

Ann was still agitated and noisy when awake. Not much more than a week into her new residence, the rest home manager was expressing concern that Ann was upsetting other residents with her distress. Ann was, I'm sure, agitated for a *number* of reasons. Looking back, we know that she found her seating arrangements uncomfortable. She became frustrated at being unable to communicate. She hated being sedated. Very importantly, she knew when she was due to urinate or have a bowel motion. Add to this that she was left alone in a small room all day — and we had a recipe for unhappiness.

To further add to her distress — once having to soil herself, she well knew that her incontinence pads were dirty. Rest home practice works around a daily ration of incontinence pads, despite them often claiming otherwise. This leads to leaving residents with soiled pads for some time. To be fair, the pads are very good, keeping the skin dry. Many residents also seem to be unaware of a soiled pad, a sort of blessing.

Ann well knew of any soiling though. During her times in various rest homes, Ann was often left with a soiled pad for some time: The caregivers seemed to feel that, once a pad has been changed, nothing needs be checked for the next couple of hours. If you should be so inconvenient as to soil your pad just after it is changed, good luck — you're stuck with it until the next check! Possibly in as little as two hours, if you're lucky.

On the positive side, the rest home GP had studied animal husbandry. He'd also done some post graduate research in the area before deciding that medicine would lead to a more useful and lucrative career. In addition, he had interests in hyperbaric oxygen therapy so was clearly of a broad-minded bent. To further encourage me, his base medical practice was in a poorer part of town with a refreshingly cosmopolitan team of doctors.

Prior to Ann moving to the rest home, I'd enquired whether the doctor would cooperate with Ann's treatment as recommended by Dr Dave. "Yes", I was told.

My first meeting with the doctor was … a pleasant surprise! By this stage, I had a standard spiel with supporting documents prepared. Working on the assumption that the likely response was somewhere between deep suspicion and outright hostility, I was astounded when the doctor cut me short. He'd already read the documentation. His comment: "I can't see that this would do any harm — could possibly do some good."

A program of detoxification and reduction of sedation was initiated. The detoxification regime was, unfortunately, still charcoal based. Not so effective. I administered Shoemaker's recommended brain healing VIP spray as often as I could, still well below what was required.

Ann's condition at this point was stable. She passed the point where the consulting neurologist had prophesied her almost certain demise. A major milestone.

A storm struck in April, cutting power to Ann's rest home. The backup generator was only able to supply power to the rest home's kitchen and public spaces. Whilst many residents were in a lounge by the fire, Ann was left alone in her room.

I arrived in the early afternoon for my daily visit, a full twelve hours after the rest home lost power. Ann was sitting alone in a freezing, unlit room, bare-footed, a light throw over her legs and a very light top. She was fortunately so sedated at this point that she didn't appear to be aware of how cold she had become. Staff complied immediately — after some very weak excuses — with my demands that she be adequately covered.

Things jogged along at the rest home for the balance of April. I worked very hard to help reduce Ann's distress and mitigate the disturbance created by her agitation. This included my accessing some industrial sound-deadening blankets to hang in her room. Ann was unhappy, not eating very well, but no longer deteriorating. However, her weight had become worryingly low: around 40kg (88lb). Even when very fit, Ann had never dropped below 55kg (120lb).

One morning, early in May 2018, I received an urgent call from the rest home: Ann had experienced a number of seizures which the rest home felt were probably the result of a stroke. I rushed to the rest home and witnessed the last of these seizures.

For the previous two or three years, Ann, when cold, would experience brief full body spasms. I had always successfully ended these by warming her up. Ann's seizure started with exactly the same spasm, progressing into a full seizure, her face going blue as she stopped breathing. Scary to watch and no doubt distressing to her.

Both Ann and the room were very cold. I'd earlier signed a "Do not Resuscitate" order in the event of a major cardiac or cerebral event. Further agreements signed indicated that in the above event, she would not be hospitalised for preventative intervention.

The fact that I had specified that such events were to be of a catastrophic nature, seemed to have been lost. The rest home manager had determined that this was the "end run" for Ann and that they should retain her until her — deemed soon to be —passing.

I instead insisted that Ann be hospitalised. Ann was transferred to the nearest public hospital, Waitakere Hospital in West Auckland. The journey towards Ann's recovery finally began.

Chapter 9

The Treatment Journey, Part 2

Ann makes a surprising and rapid improvement.
We find out what works. The battle continues…

Ann's supply of VIP nasal spray was extremely expensive. According to Shoemaker, the spray was critical to Ann's brain function recovery. In January 2018 a local pharmaceutical compounding company had accessed the drug for Ann, at huge expense - a six-week supply priced out at NZ$6,500 (USD$4,300).

I accepted the high price, since it was very important that Ann receive the medication as soon as possible, although this cost was clearly not sustainable. Fortunately some internet research had indicated the drug was available much more cheaply elsewhere.

I eventually tracked down a compounding laboratory in Australia who could supply the same amount of the drug for NZ$300 (USD$200). However, I would need an Australian medical prescription to order the drug. The laboratory recommend that I contact Lotus Holistic Medicine in Maroochydore, Queensland, Australia.

6. Pete's Sixth Rule for Beating Alzheimer's

Get what you need. Once you know what it is you require, it will always turn up... exactly when you need it.

Upon reviewing Lotus' website, I realised I had found exactly the people I needed. Dr Sandeep Gupta, the lead practitioner was a specialist in Lyme-related CIRS. Dr Gupta consulted internationally with a lot of his work involving supporting CIRS patients on the eastern seaboard of the USA and Canada.

Dr Rashmi Cabena had just joined the practice. She'd just moved to the area from Melbourne, Australia. Her particular expertise was the treatment of metals toxicity and mineral deficiencies.

She became Ann's practitioner in February 2018 and remains a huge contributor to Ann's continuing improvement. Dr Cabena helped us establish a more rounded regime, with some mineral supplementation added to assist with what she felt to be most likely deficiencies.

The key recommendation was that Ann have tissue testing to check both her levels of essential minerals and to explore possible toxicity issues. Dr Cabena told me that tissue sampling could reveal the existence of compounds that may not show up in blood testing.

Fortunately, a new non-invasive technology, the Oligoscan had recently become available. The test was simple and quick. A telephone headset- sized device was held on different parts of Ann's hand four or five times as directed by the attached laptop computer: The device fired a low intensity laser beam into the hand, then read the wavelengths of the reflected light.

An Oligoscan is a spectrophotometer. For those of you who did high school chemistry, you'll possibly remember your lessons on the light signatures of different chemicals. Never having studied chemistry, I gave myself a quick lesson to help understand the technology.

Spectrophotometry is used widely in: chemistry; pharmacy; environmental science; food processing; biology; medicine; materials/chemical engineering; and other fields. The Oligoscan device is generally used to track both essential mineral levels and toxic metal levels in real time. The advantages being, not only initial detection of the levels, but tracking the effectiveness of treatments.

What we found:

Ann was both low on essential minerals, and had very high levels of metals toxicity, aluminium and mercury being notable. Dr Cabena suggested that these levels alone would have compromised Ann's immune system. Add the CIRS genetic susceptibility, and we had a serious problem just waiting to happen.

Finally we had a comprehensive picture of Ann's challenges, plus a practitioner with some good ideas and the necessary experience, to advance Ann's recovery.

However, we were not out of the woods yet. At this stage it was still early May 2018. Ann had just been admitted to Waitakere Hospital.

It was 10pm and she hadn't had any of her many medications for thirty hours. She was highly distressed, especially as most of her drugs are reported to have habit-forming characteristics. Morphine being possibly the worst.

The attending ward doctor looked at Ann's chart of medications, supplied by the rest home. He noted the morphine, supposedly prescribed for pain. I told him, "no more morphine": It had clearly been a major component in Ann's stupefied waking state.

During Ann's earlier stay at the psychiatric wing at North Shore Hospital, each failed drug intervention gave rise to more drugs. Ann's 'date rape'-type experience being an example. Ann's agitation during handling had lead our cloth-eared friends, the psychiatrists, to assume Ann was experiencing pain. Their answer? Heavy daily dosages of morphine. The result? No change. At one point an increased dosage led to an immediate increase in agitation. Reduction of the dosage — at my request — achieved a decrease in agitation.

So, we achieved a cessation of the morphine. The result — no increase in agitation and Ann was immediately much more aware when awake. Similarly, large doses of paracetamol were ceased. A dose of another anti-psychotic drug, also part of Ann's regime, settled her down.

The next day was to be a pleasant revelation... The hospital attending physician arrived with her bevy of 'apprentice' doctors, three house registrars. I met them clutching my standard package of information, including Ann's notes from Dr Dave and the CIRS test results. I was expecting the normal response which, experience had taught me, could range from guarded acceptance to outright disparagement.

The physician read Ann's CIRS test results. Upon viewing the interpretative accompanying notes, she said to the registrars, "I want you to listen to this. This is where medicine is going."

My jaw dropped. Was this the start of a new phase? Had we broken through the resistance at last? What then followed was three weeks of Ann being properly cared for with a well-monitored reduction of the remaining medications.

Ann's care regime crossed over from palliative to rehabilitative. An immediate result was assessment by the hospital occupational therapy team. This lead to

Ann receiving a specialist mobility chair two months later.

I continued to prepare food for Ann: Each day I would take in lunch and dinner. The hospital dieticians had no idea of what comprised a ketogenic diet, let alone awareness of the well-documented inability of an Alzheimer's brain to effectively obtain energy from glucose.

Where had these people had been for the last twenty years as the world awakened to the damage being wrought by the grain-based food pyramid?

I felt vindicated in my efforts over the past year. Many of the ward nurses took the trouble to read Ann's background notes that I'd supplied. To be approached by a nurse and receive positive comments on Ann's treatment protocols, was heartening indeed. To this day, the physician and I correspond. More than once she has taken time from her busy schedule to phone me to discuss issues I have raised.

During the time at Waitakere Hospital, I set about finding a rest home that could comply with Ann's treatment requirements — as outlined by Dr Dave and Dr Cabena.

I was also concerned that we start physical rehabilitation as Ann's arms and legs were badly wasted by over nine months of zero activity. In addition, and more worrying, her arm and leg tendons were showing signs of shrinkage — if left untreated, an irreversible condition.

I located an upmarket rest home which boasted great facilities including a hydrotherapy pool and a gym. I was assured that Ann's agitation wouldn't be an issue. Nor would meeting her ketogenic dietary requirements. Staffing levels were higher than normal for the sector, care was superior, the manager assured me.

The rest home didn't have a vacancy. We would have to wait. The hospital needed Ann's bed as winter, the busiest season, approached. I needed to find an interim rest home to care for Ann.

The lessons were piling up:

7. Pete's Seventh Rule for Beating Alzheimer's

Prioritise quality care over impressive surroundings.

There is often an inverse relationship between the quality of the surroundings and the quality of rest home care.

It was a year since Ann went into care. This was her sixth rest home placement. She'd had four hospital admissions.

The interim rest home was an offence to my middle class sensitivities. Over the years we had either renovated or built all our homes. We were used to having control over our surroundings. We also liked them to be freshly decorated with the latest facilities.

The interim rest home was none of the above.

The place had been built on a tight budget twenty years previously, and —frankly — it showed. Cheap surfaces and wall coverings were showing the effects of 20 year's hard use.

The resident's kitchen-dining area was run-down: Cabinetry had loose edges, doubtless harbouring germs; the dishwasher was an old budget model with the internal fittings falling apart; opening the kitchen drawers was a ... squirmy experience; cutlery and linen were short; food handling hygiene less than stellar — sticky hands the result of a a foray into the area.

The place failed the 'urine test': The hallways smelt of pee.

However, the standard of care and the contentment of the residents belied the above appearances.

I had now assembled the complex requirements to fully implement Ann's treatment plan as jointly established by Dr Dave and Dr Cabena. A program involving up to six daily administrations of a complex array of supplements and medications. Added to this were the further requirements of Ann's behaviour and comfort medication regime. Fortunately much reduced.

The rest home readily agreed to all of the above. The attending GP was cooperative and indicating an interest in further reducing Ann's sedative medications.

Furthermore, the rest home chef spent two hours with me. As with so many new migrants, her level of education and skill well exceeded her position. After some explanation, she clearly understood Ann's dietary requirements and the reasoning behind them. Her interpretation of Ann's needs lead to one of the remarkable changes wrought in Ann's two weeks at the rest home.

On the 22nd May 2018, Ann arrived by ambulance at the rest home. She was often agitated when awake. She was eating, but not enthusiastically — she weighed 40kg (88lb). She was barely communicating, and only at a very basic level.

For the first time we were able to fully implement her treatments for both the CIRS and metals toxicity issues. We were also able to address her mineral deficiencies. The kitchen was able to provide appropriate food.

A 'miracle' happened - another one!

Immediately, Ann was eating enthusiastically. In the words of our oldest son she was 'inhaling' a normal diet — no more mush or pureed food.

Within ten days she was able to tell the nurses who I was when I was not present. "Who is your husband?" asked the nurses. "Peter," was the reply.

One day, I heard her calling out as I arrived. The nurses told me she had been asking "Where are the boys?" — being Ann's brother Mike, and his partner John, who had visited two days previously.

Ann was quiet, appeared to be taking a lot of interest in her surroundings, and was talking to the nurses in full, if simple, sentences. She was quiet when handled, bearing out my long-held suspicion that her agitation was a result of her not fully understanding what was happening.

A friend with forty-five years' experience in dealing with disabled people had been periodically observing Ann whilst visiting Auckland on business. Amongst his many skills was a deep understanding of communication abilities in disabled people.

He was stunned at the progress Ann had made in 4 weeks, spanning her time at the hospital and a week at the rest home.

His words: "If you tried to tell me that Ann had made this much progress, I would not have believed you."

This was not to last.

Chapter 10

An Attempted Takeover

The medical profession fight to retain control of Ann's treatment

Looking back on the journey, and with the wisdom of hindsight, I realise that I made one of the biggest errors of Ann's journey.

As you'll find when your level of knowledge of rises and you become an expert in the needs of your loved one, you'll get increasing resistance from medical professionals. They'll be unwilling to accept that you may — in a specific and impassioned area in which the personal stakes are high —- know more than they do.

Over a four-week period spanning Ann's time at the hospital and her temporary rest home placement, I had been negotiating her move to the upmarket rest home mentioned in the last chapter. The home was situated in the rural west of Auckland. Large, near new, well appointed with attractive gardens and an ambience more like an hotel than a rest home. All appearances were that Ann would have the perfect home to continue her recovery. The gym, and particularly the hydrotherapy pool, would be a great bonus.

I supplied a lot of information regarding Ann's condition and the recommended treatments. I met with the clinical director and the nurse manager - a long meeting to go through the details of Ann's condition and the treatments required.

At this stage, Dr Cabena had assumed full control of Ann's treatment program, with Dr Dave keeping an overview.

All was agreeable, with much goodwill and interest being expressed by the meeting participants. The rest home had four weeks to contact former carers to get a professional view of her condition and behaviours.

Ann moved to the rest home early June 2018. What followed was 5 weeks of hell. The rest home management showed themselves to be anything *but* caring or pleasant. In contrast the staff, as always, were fantastic.

Another lesson, another guiding principle:

8. Pete's Eighth Rule for Beating Alzheimer's

Look *past* the PR. Privately owned rest homes are run for profit. Difficult residents are a nuisance.

All protestations about being 'caring' are PR (Public Relations) fluff to be taken with a grain of salt.

Occasional exceptions to the rule? See Rule Seven.

The rest home catering staff stepped up to the plate. Despite the manager's assurances, the staff were blank when asked about preparing Ann a ketogenic diet. We worked on this and Ann was quickly fed delicious, nutritious food — and in large quantities, as her now-voracious appetite demanded.

Unfortunately the diet was rich in dairy food, not recommended as it is known to aid inflammation. Ann quickly developed colic, the result being severe pain after eating. She became severely agitated after her meals.

In addition, Ann's bowels were now very active, as was her urinary tract, given that she was drinking the large quantities of fluids recommended by Dr Cabena. Further complications started to arise as Ann's earlier lucid periods strongly suggested she knew when she was about to toilet. She clearly knew when she *had*. Leaving her, even in a lightly soiled incontinence pad, was distressing for her. And not just mentally so: She quickly developed a severe rash — sometimes bleeding — across her anal and vaginal areas.

So, Ann was soon in severe discomfort. She had gained strength and was still gaining weight. Her lungs were good — always good, she sang at high school operas without a microphone. She couldn't express herself as the distress had caused her a regression in her communication skills. Her only means of expression? To scream. Loudly.

I had always made myself available to Ann's rest homes when needed. Her life insurance payout had enabled me to make caring for Ann my full-time job ... for a while at least. I told the rest home to notify me if Ann became agitated and noisy: I came at once if the problem occurred outside my normal hours of daily attendance.

I spent several evenings with Ann screaming. Eventually, sedation and exhaustion would defeat her and she would fall asleep. During these periods we were moved to an isolated part of the facility. Unsurprisingly, Ann's agitation was upsetting the other residents.

No means were provided to summon either nurses or caregivers. Staff were issued with earplugs, though neither Ann or I were. Despite my strong suspicion that Ann was suffering severe colic, no effective measures were taken at any time during her stay. I repeatedly asked for the rest home doctor to treat the colic (a condition later confirmed when she went to hospital).

At the end of the first week, I attended a meeting with medical staff, including the clinical director and the rest home doctor. The term 'possible failed admission' was raised by the clinical director. When I challenged this, a quick backdown occurred — to my face at least.

Up to this point, the rest home nursing staff were administering all the medications and supplements recommended by Dr Cabena. This was not to last.

Over the next two weeks, a process similar to a 'constructive dismissal' began. Constructive dismissal is a term used to describe an employer's attempts to dismiss unwanted staff without due process. It involves inventing a series of 'problems' which lead to an inevitable parting of the ways. A practice deservedly penalised in employment law.

Suddenly, there were 'ethical' reasons preventing the nurses from administering Ann's treatments. I was told nursing staff were concerned that their professional registrations were at risk. I checked — the nurses were bemused as they had not expressed any such concerns.

I worked very hard to make Ann's residence work. I offered to soundproof her room at our expense: An offer not taken up. Shortly thereafter, Ann was evicted, given three week's notice. The clinical manager and rest home manager showed themselves to have a truly nasty streak.

As I write, we are in the process of a legal mediation process to address extra costs. Some were paid, some were not, such as a premium of $50 per day charged by the home above the government's already substantial daily payment.

Typically a premium is charged when high-value extra services are provided. My contention was that Ann's basic care was deficient and agreed treatments were withdrawn. The much-vaunted higher staffing ratios were, in Ann's case, meaningless: it simply wasn't reflected in her standard of care.

In addition, a vital service that had led me to placing Ann in the home was absent: The hydrotherapy pool had become ornamental — the pumps being out of action and unlikely to be fixed for some time. This, I was told only *after* Ann's admission. And no sign of any physiotherapy, another item promised at our pre-admission meeting.

The money involved is relatively minor, but the principle isn't. In addition I wanted to ensure the rest home's performance was widely publicised. *Consumer*, New Zealand's not-for-profit consumer rights organisation, watches the Care industry with interest. Poor rest home performance has become a major concern to their members. *Consumer* promises to report to their membership on the mediation, such reports invariably finding their way into national NZ media.

Amongst other imagined transgressions, apparently I was intimidating staff. The only staff I appeared to challenge — the nurses were always wonderful — were the centre's manager and clinical manager.

Every day, as Lexus and I walked to Ann's room I had several chats with the catering staff, caregivers, nurses and cleaning staff. All pleasant and friendly. I would like to think my sunny personality was the cause, however, being Lexus' media assistant, I *well* knew why the conversations started! The day we left, two of the 'intimidated' staff spontaneously hugged me as I made our farewells and thanked them for their help.

As for the management, they did find me intimidating, and deservedly so. I was *determined* that their obscene behaviour would be exposed and set about making sure the government funding authorities knew of our experiences. Much of the rest home funding came via government-provided subsidies, on behalf of many residents.

By this time, the funding authorities had intervened. Senior staffers for both rest home placements and social work became involved. In typical fashion, the rest home management had done their best to paint me as being obsessive and unreasonable.

This endeavour was aided by their supplying an attending community dementia nurse with a good body of disinformation about my 'unreasonable' demands. They also did their best to discredit Ann's medical advisors and their advice. An effective 'white anting', to use a political term.

Drawing on her many years experience of comprehensive failure to improve the prospects of the Alzheimer's sufferers she had attended, the dementia nurse circulated a report backing the rest home's position. It was as though we should collectively believe that Ann's medical advisors knew nothing compared to this 'expert'. Possessing a vaguely specified postgraduate qualification in Dementia, this woman felt she could dismiss all the information supplied which came from some of the world's best practitioners in their fields.

The nurse's report became a problem — up until I obtained a copy. As this woman clearly felt she knew best, she set about trying to take away my legal power over Ann's welfare. Ann had given me, whilst still able, an Enduring Power of Attorney over her physical welfare, her brother being the back-up in the event of my incapacity. Our daughter held Power of Attorney over Ann's financial and property affairs.

Threats were made to legally challenge my Power of Attorney. My daughter received a phone call from this woman telling her that the public health authorities were on the verge of doing so. She intimated that this would be relatively easy and quick. We would lose control over Ann's welfare. Understandably, our children were very upset.

The message was loud and clear: "If your father doesn't bow to our recommendations, we'll take over. You'll have no say in Ann's welfare." "And it's easy to do." My family well knew what that would mean. They would lose their mother, and in a very short time.

I took legal advice from our long-time lawyer:

No, the courts would not just roll over on this. Their view of Ann's welfare and the extensive expertise behind her treatment program, would be filtered in an unbiased fashion. Clearly, I had been acting in Ann's best interests, driven by the best advice I could find.

Ann's backup attorney is her brother. He was in complete agreement with what I'd done, making it pretty much impossible to overturn our control of Ann's care.

9. Pete's Ninth Rule for Beating Alzheimer's

Be on guard. Rather than admit they may have it wrong, conventional carers will often stop at nothing to obstruct your loved one's treatment.

They would far rather have a person die than challenge their superstition that Alzheimer's is untreatable.

This is a war... Make no mistake.

Failure leads to death.

The lowest point of the whole experience (yes, it does get lower) was the rest home doctor's proposal to euthanise Ann.

A few days before Ann's departure from the rest home, the doctor came in after-hours to visit. A surprise as he had been avoiding me for some time.

The following discussion was carried out in Ann's presence and went thus:

- I'm a doctor, you're not. How dare you tell me my job.

- Ann has advanced terminal dementia and will die soon. None of Bredesen's work succeeded with later stage patients (true, but not necessarily so for CIRS).

- We should keep her at the rest home and heavily sedate her so she isn't distressed or noisy.

- The sedation will suppress her appetite which will weaken her (she'd been gaining weight for 6 weeks at this point).

- The sedation will cause her to contract aspiration pneumonia as she inhales food or drink, causing her to die.

All done — dust off your hands, Ann's dead. Everyone's happy, the "Alzheimer's Can't be Cured" gravy train rolls on ...

No-one has to think, or have doubts about the ethics of *deliberately* ignoring the *growing* body of well-documented research. Research telling them they're sending many people to an unnecessary, early death.

During this discussion, Ann was lying in her bed screaming. The doctor left in frustration at my refusal to 'listen to good sense'. Ann stops. He came back. Ann started screaming again:

She'd made her feelings clear

10. Pete's Tenth Rule for Rule for Beating Alzheimer's

Never give up. An Alzheimer's patient will fall under the care of professionals who are convinced there is no hope of improvement or survival.

They will rank life no higher than a family pet, offering an organised demise with no right of reply.

Prepare for battle with the determination and drive of Winston Churchill.

The sorry saga at the upmarket rest home drew to a close... I had senior funding authority staff assisting with finding a suitable rest home placement. They were starting to understand that I was not being unreasonable in my requirements for Ann's care.

Moves were underway to reclaim extra charges from the rest home. More importantly, publicity will accompany the mediation process. Hopefully the community dementia nurse is learning that there are boundaries that shouldn't be crossed - moves are afoot to have her censured by senior managers. She's dangerously incompetent and needs to be controlled.

The rest home, though, is of the mistaken impression that a problem has disappeared.

Ann's emotional state had deteriorated as had her apparent cognitive state. She had severe colic pain and was generally very unhappy. We'd lost a lot of progress.

Ann was moved to a geriatric rehabilitation unit at North Shore Hospital.

Chapter 11

The Treatment Journey: Part 3

**Ann is treated properly for her physical ailments.
A step backwards becomes a step forwards**

Within two hours of Ann's admission to hospital, nursing staff picked up that she was experiencing extreme gut pain. They liaised with the ward geriatrician who prescribed an injectable drug specifically for cramping pain. Immediately, Ann was more comfortable.

Colic is a word we bandy around without fully understanding how painful it can be. Fortunately, for my understanding of the problem, I'd experienced it two years previously: I'd spent eight days in the same hospital as a result of a ruptured appendix. The appendix was removed via keyhole surgery. One of the surgeons told me there had been a lot of cleaning up required — my intestines had been significantly disturbed.

Four days of intense pain followed. Now, I dislike pain medications. During my several experiences in hospital, usually for injuries, I'd learned to get off them very quickly. Not so with the colic — injected morphine *barely managed* the pain.

Why had the rest home not acted in the five weeks she was with them? I will never know. Thank goodness we'd left them behind.

Shortly after Ann's admission, two specialist occupational therapists arrived to deliver and fit Ann's new mobility chair. Prior to this, Ann had been seated in an electric LazyBoy. Not ideal when you have no ability to reposition yourself when uncomfortable. Shifting around in a chair to get comfortable is something that we just take for granted.

Immediately, Ann was more comfortable and felt secure when seated, naturally leading to her having more time out of bed. But when I arrived one day, shortly after the arrival of the chair, Ann was clearly very agitated — a nurse had mistakenly thought Ann would be more comfortable in her LazyBoy. We quickly shifted Ann to her new mobility chair. She settled immediately, the LazyBoy went into retirement. Ann had made her opinion known.

At this point Ann's CIRS treatment had collapsed.

A key requirement was the detoxification regime, recommended and well-documented by Dr Shoemaker. Past experience had shown this to be vital. In both instances where we'd managed to get the detoxification protocol fully in place, Ann's condition *had* improved, hugely.

Despite the very good care Ann received at the hospital, she continued to be agitated. After two weeks, I began to administer her detox treatments. Practically it was impossible to achieve more than two dosages a day, often only a few hours apart.

The recommendation was three times daily, away from food or medication. Timing was crucial, this was a physical cleansing of biotoxins produced by Ann's CIRS. Effective administration required the dosages to be spread from early morning to late evening.

The ward geriatrician was ... resistant. With the surety of the ill-informed, she told me that she did not believe that CIRS caused Alzheimer's. However, she did take the trouble to read the volumes of supplied literature. She was concerned that the Cholestyramine recommended by Shoemaker could cause complications.

Over the second week of Ann's admission, I bombarded the geriatrician with research papers documenting both the efficacy and benign nature of the drug.

Finally, she relented. The ward took over the administration of the detox regime, it was now spread from 7 am to 9 pm.

Ann then began a gradual improvement which continues to this day. Over the remaining three weeks at the hospital, Ann began to regain function, becoming less agitated. When finally agitated, she called out rather than screamed. She began to address nurses by name — all the staff seemed amazed at her progress.

During Ann's time in the hospital, I worked closely with the funding authority's aforementioned social worker and rest home placement specialist.

After considerable research and negotiation, the decision was made to move Ann back to the rest home where she had done so well in May of this year of writing, 2018. The rest home where, in two short weeks, Ann had improved so much.

As I write, Ann has been there two days.

Already a marked improvement: Her situational sedation regime has all but disappeared; the rest home is preferring to investigate the causes of Ann's distress, rather than sedate her. Their tolerance for disruption being much higher than a hospital ward, understandably.

Last night, I fed her dinner. As has been her habit, she was agitated after her meal. A situation generally resulting in sedation at the hospital. The agitation was of low intensity and short lived. No sedation required.

Ann's communication has improved. Her awareness has improved.

Why?

It's hard to tell. Certainly, Ann doesn't like being in hospital. When giving birth to our three children, she couldn't leave hospital fast enough — an overnight stay was her limit.

The battles come and go, some won, some lost — but the war against the enemy at the gate, is ongoing.

Afterword

Where to now?

We've turned the tide. What about you?

Before you start a war, you need to identify the enemy. In this case, several enemies:

- The symptoms and their associated causes

- A medical establishment committed to an impossibly-naïve negative position. Ready to let people die rather than admit they have it wrong

- A 'caregiving' juggernaut which is profiting hugely from providing palliative care to those whom they should be healing

The first stage of victory is to turn the tide. Stop the enemy's advance, weaken its resistance and, in time, start to attack. We are now in the early stages of our attack, in the face of huge opposition from those who should be our allies.

Arrest and reversal of Ann's symptoms? This is something we've already achieved. A full cure is something we can't achieve with the weapons available. Yet. We know that Ann's future welfare will require ongoing interventions. Our new normal will continue to require huge efforts to maintain and improve Ann's state.

I'm often asked where I think this is all going. I have no idea. We are in uncharted territory. Ann is one of the first people in the world to survive diagnosed end-stage terminal Alzheimer's.

What will Ann's future look like? Again, an unknown. What functions she'll recover is impossible to predict. Time will tell. She could, as both her parents have done, live another 30 years. She could spend those 30 years as a severely disabled person. Or not.

As I write, the possibility of taking her home has become real. An impossible dream a few weeks ago, is now becoming an action plan. I'm now convinced that Ann will do better, with supporting care, at home.

The End

For Now

Appendix I

What about you?

Likely you're reading this because you have a family member that is showing worrying symptoms. Where do you start?

First Step:

Gird your loins.

This is not for the faint-hearted. This is war, losing is not an option. Here's the starting point:

- How much do you love this person?

- How deep is your commitment?

Is it total or conditional. 'Til Death do us part' or 'Til Death do us part as long as it's convenient'? Your commitment may have been stated in other ways but needs to be as deep.

A message for my fellow males: Most of you dump your partners in a rest home and run. I'm an outlier, a male caring for a female partner. Time to take a 'Harden the Heck up Pill' and step up. I mean it. Twice as many women develop Alzheimer's symptoms as men do. The vast majority of people involved in going the extra mile for their partners are women. Do the numbers...

Second Step:

Arm yourself with knowledge.

This will take time and effort. It will be worth it. Strength comes from knowledge and commitment. Without both factors, you will fail. Appendix 2 will give you some places to start.

Third Step:

Do *something* today:

- **Start with diet**
    - ✓ Ditch starchy and sugary foods
    - ✓ Alcohol has to go.
    - ✓ Find out what a ketogenic diet is and implement it.
    - ✓ Introduce coconut oil into your diet.
- **Exercise daily**

    … as much as is possible.
- **Stay mentally stimulated**
    - ✓ Turn off the TV
    - ✓ Watch Ted talks on your computer instead
- **Have fun!**
    - ✓ Listen to music
    - ✓ Watch comedy
    - ✓ Laugh
    - ✓ Cuddle…a lot

Fourth Step:

Look for help of the right sort

This will most likely exclude your doctor or neurologist. They will break your heart and destroy all hope.

They will know nothing of the great research and successful treatment being pioneered. Their default position will be that "Alzheimer's is incurable". "Cure" meaning a magic pill. Stupidly naïve when even some understanding of the problem is gained. 25 years of failed drug trials would signal something to most people. Not so this group.

Fifth Step

Talk to the right people

With all enterprises, success has a lot to do with the company you keep. You'll meet many naysayers. Your job is not to proselytise, it's to win. When you're winning, let people know — you'll help save lives.

Alzheimer's support associations are run by well-meaning, caring people. Unfortunately the whole flavour is of administering care to the doomed. Not a healthy milieu to be near. Unless you really feel the need of their support, they're probably best avoided.

And a final word

Earlier I mentioned the fortuitous arrival of the right help exactly when it's needed.

Ann and I have always been *pragmatists* — not at all religious.

Experience has shown that, unfailingly, the right help arrives at the right time. Different groups attribute this to different entities. Religious people speak of the power of prayer. Others talk of the 'Quantum Effect'. There are many theories. I have no position — apart from *knowing* that it works.

What I do also know, is that you must be aware of what you need so that you'll recognise it when it arrives.

Hopefully, this book will be that needed arrival for you.

Appendix 2

Resources

**Here follow some good places
to find your first weapons**

Start here ...

Go to www.svhi.com

Search "Dr Dale Bredesen"

An address by Dr Dale Bredesen, November 17th 2016, to the Silicon Valley Health Institute. A plain language explanation of his research and diagnostic methodology. Bredesen's work quite literally saved Ann's life.

For a good explanation of the Bredesen Protocol in practice, and real life examples:

www.endalzheimers.com.au

This website will introduce you to Ann's Bredesen Doctor, Dr Dave Jenkins. Dr Dave kindly agreed to work with us despite Ann being outside of the normal parameters for the Bredesen Protocol.

Dr Dave can take direct credit for saving Ann's life. Without his dedication, we would have never found out that Ann has CIRS

More ...

Read Dr Bredesen's excellent book:

The End of Alzheimer's: The First Programme to Prevent and Reverse the Cognitive Decline of Dementia

(Available from Amazon in Kindle and paperback formats)

...

A very good background to the whole nutrition side of the equation:

Alzheimer's Disease: What if There Was a Cure: The Story of Ketones

- Dr Mary Newport

(Available from Amazon in Kindle and paperback formats)

Dr Newport is publishing a new book, due February 2019:

The Complete Book of Ketones: A Practical Guide to Ketogenic Diets and Ketone Supplements

...

An excellent and comprehensive book on the importance of correct diet for good health and rehabilitation:

Fat for Fuel: A Revolutionary Diet to Combat Cancer, Boost Brain Power, and Increase Your Energy

- Dr Joseph Mercola

(Available from Amazon in Kindle and paperback formats)

...

Specifically for Ann's particular condition…

Go to www.ncbi.nim.nih.gov

Search: "Inhalational Alzheimer's Disease: an Unrecognised—and Treatable—Epidemic",

(Dr Dale Bredesen)

This is a paper on "Inhalational Alzheimer's" from Dr Bredesen, containing a concise explanation of Bredesen's protocol and Ann's specific issues.

If you have my low level of medical knowledge, stick to the first couple of pages.

...

Finally, again for Ann's specific condition (most CIRS is caused by leaky buildings):

Google: "Surviving Mould Downunder"

(Dr Sandeep Gupta)

This is a practical guide with a very good explanation of CIRS, by Dr Sandeep Gupta.

Dr Gupta is the lead practitioner at Lotus Holistic Medicine. Dr Rashmi Cabena is his associate.

Made in the USA
Columbia, SC
09 February 2020

87703285R00076